Becoming a Health Coach

Becoming a Health Coach

Jules Hawthorne

Contents

1

Introduction to Health Coaching

Have you been curious about health coaching? Health coaching is a gentle, personal exploration that moves people from where they are to where they want to be in their life. Health coaching is a relatively new profession as it has been around for 30 years, but it has drastically increased in popularity over the past 20 years in the United States. With that, now is a perfect opportunity to become a health coach. Integrative wellness is becoming a new standard when it comes to healthcare, and hiring a health coach is on the rise. Integrative wellness is the physical, emotional, spiritual, and mental way of looking at the human species. This is the mindset and way of life our practitioners use to help enrich the lives of all clients that come in.

Whether you begin the path to become a health coach or want to master the integrative wellness side of the human body, if you are ready to help others in their journey and evolve as your own person then this is 100% for you. Being a health coach is not just a new career that will give you a better paycheck, it is a new way of life. A health coach is a guide and mentor who empowers clients to take responsibility for their own health and supports them in making sustainable changes to their lives. The idea is to stimulate a person and other practitioners to reach the maximum true potential and potential success in their career path. In addition, it can be working with the patient and referral source to ensure they are working with their collective healthcare team in the best possible way to achieve maximum outcomes for everyone involved.

Defining Health Coaching

Health coaching, in particular, is a profession that offers support by using what is known in the world of somatics as an "inside-out" approach. This means that coaches trust that the people they're coaching know best about what is right for them. Because it is based on this principle, health coaching can be seen as a universal tool to help us connect with our most basic knowledge - what it feels like to be ourselves. This knowledge can be accessed just as easily by someone with a master's degree as by an eight-year-old child, a person with many chronic health conditions just as easily as someone who feels fit. After all, we are each the best subjects for the fascinating study of what it's like to be an embodied being.

Almost every aspect of what is meant by health can be deeply emotional, as your own stories have perhaps revealed to you. So much so that the parameters that make up health can seem at times as fine as the air. A definition of health would certainly include the fact that it's a sense of feeling well in body, mind, and spirit made real in countless aspects of daily life - interpersonal relationships, work, sexuality. I define health coaching, therefore, as a therapeutic conversation that is informed by concepts of belief about health, what has created health in your life in the past and may still be creating health now, focused in the present, and carries an awareness of both the miracle and limitations of being human. The conversation is collaborative and respectful, never coercive. In the field of integrative medicine, this kind of coaching respects that health outcomes have as much to do with the live context of a person as with their "objective" medical condition.

The Role of a Health Coach

Health coaches support individuals to move beyond obstacles and self-imposed barriers to integrating new lifestyle behaviors. A health coach is not an old-fashioned "teacher" or "instructor." Instead, a coach works together with another person to create a process that encourages the clarification of the individual's personal values and the development of sustainable goals to move forward to new levels of whole-person wellness. Along the way, the coach supports processes that build enthusiasm and positive attitudes towards well-being that also enhance health.

Health coaches also must be prepared to work effectively with healthcare professionals. This involves being able to understand the language, medical protocols, clinical time and work pressures, and other factors in healthcare. This is likely to be part of the required training in your health coach program. Always check for this though. It will help you move into partnerships with healthcare and achieve your career goals. Health coaches support individuals to develop and sustain healthful new habits that are grounded in integrative solutions for well-being. This aspect is the primary focus for health coach education. Integrative wellness aligns with and assists patients/clients to build and sustain well-being in integrative healthcare settings and practices as well.

Benefits of Integrative Wellness

Striving to include one's well-being in the plethora of decisions we make involves a shift from the traditional, reactive model of healthcare to a more proactive approach. A holistic approach to health encompasses a broad range of behaviors, attitudes, ideals, and opportunities. It is not limited to one's diet, but may also incorporate activities such as emotional healing and counseling, physical activity and brain-boosting exercises, rest, and rejuvenation.

Issues can be anticipated and safeguarded from as a result of such approaches, as well as having a substantial impact on our emotional, psychological, and physical well-being. Unity infant, age is not a bad factor any longer gi oh all ay affected, developing inhabitants are committed to taking account of their bodily, cognitive, and psychological well-being by building more health in their lives as they develop and develop from an early stage. As an offshoot, we also find a rise in leaders dedicated to doing the same for themselves. The impacts of some improvement being eternally smoothed calm on pulp appear to be a retreat from changed hack and coracle orientation and health placement in some orbits. Reliable techniques are improbable to be an actual exploration of the anticipated wretchedness of see anguish; rather, they are examination care and factors. Accomplishment of such propositions for each girl would earnestly congregate a final moderator for magnification.

2

Foundations of Integrative Wellness

Psychoneuroimmunology reflects the growing understanding of the interaction between mind and body, while deepened appreciation for contextual, social, and economic factors illuminates how these may impact the expression of health. Shifts in modern metabolic disease have shown re-emerging interest in, appreciation for, and enlightenment regarding the unity of the body, central nervous system (CNS), mind, and spirit. Studies of the gut-brain axis challenge the somato-psychic separatism we inherit from the time of Descartes. A convergence of philosophy, anthropologic paleobiology, and osteopathic medicine led D.D. Palmer to posit that the correct positioning of the skeleton can lead to an optimal flow of spiritual fluids and the continuation of life. From the Māori concept of Hauora to 1950s discussions of 'full-function', the World Health Organization's conversation on health and the original mission of the National Institute of Health, a growing understanding of wellness, or the wholeness of the person, has deepened and broadened through the centuries.

Integrated health and wellness notes the need to understand and tend to all aspects of people enmeshed in the context of their communities and environs in this particular time and space configuration that we call human. So there are several foundational considerations—and one could argue that they could be considered a priori—to establish the context for anyone reading about and practicing integrative wellness. Here are the key, foundational aspects: Establish where and when we exist and the philosophical principles that provide us with the most coherent basis to discuss our approach to healthcare. Identifying and clearly stating the terminology and language we use and define the key terms that identify and help describe the principal features of our subject matter on the basis of philosophy. Define our personal core values and philosophy that we practice each day and that form the basis/markers for developing the profession.

Understanding the Mind-Body Connection

Cognition, speech, thoughts, and beliefs all share a line of communication with the seemingly physical areas of the brain, such as digestion, libido, the heartbeat, and stored memories. This mind-body connection is significant because when one of the faculties on either side is out of balance, they all are. At the most basic level, therapy is used to relieve us of physical ailments, while even the most invasive of medical treatments heavily rely on the ability of the body to heal and rejuvenate itself. Intensive training in specialized segments of healthcare is mandatory; however, Sharon's coaching method is to understand the significance of the big picture. She advises a "less is more" approach, which depends on the principle of equipping ourselves with a comprehensive, multi-disciplinary expertise with various approaches, including medical science, rather than the opposite approach of huge expertise in tiny areas.

People who are struggling with chronic digestive difficulties, or a series of diseases without any cause, or have tried a variety of solutions only to find that they are not only extremely variable when it comes to their efficacy, but also burdensome, invasive, and even counter-productive, based on the person and the situation. Protocol therapy is as divergent as the state of the art as it is the ordinary, Sharon has concluded in her practice. More and more patients, according to a recent poll, would rather struggle with their condition than have to deal with the side effects of their medication, particularly since they are underutilized in practice. Illness without a cause that is undetermined remains a pertinent cause of discomfort. Not surprisingly, she receives emails from individuals that describe fatigue as their "consistent range of feelings."

Holistic Approaches to Health and Wellbeing

Many ancient cultures in the world have developed practices that focus on approaching health from a holistic or comprehensive angle. In studying wellness now and learning about health coaching, it can be valuable to consider other methods for care that people access to help themselves feel better. These methods of care described can be called "complementary" because they are used alongside what we consider more well-established medical treatments ("alternative" methods are called such because they replace conventional or standard care). Integrative health approaches and patient-centered care are embracing alternative and complementary methods in part because these practices promise to help people get better.

Acupuncture, massage therapy, and meditation are just a few examples of different approaches to health developed as cultural knowledge throughout history. With an infusion of these and other influences, the "holistic" is an approach to health and wellbeing that takes the entire person into account during the process of care. There is a more whole-person focus with holistic and integrative health that encompasses the mind and spirit, and not just at the physical level. In some settings, the care team may bring together providers representing conventional or standard care along with those practicing and applying complementary and alternative approaches to health. These centers and professionals often operate from an alternative model of health, or what it means to "be well". Alternative therapies also consider an individual and his or her personal beliefs, strengths, and health problems within the framework of the family, community, culture, and larger social setting.

3

Nutrition and Dietary Guidelines

Nutrition and dietary guidelines are a huge portion of the content in the Integrative Nutrition curriculum. It follows the concept that "if it can be done sustainably, and if it works for you, then by all means give it a try, however there are no one-size-fits-all diets". In terms of curriculum, we begin at a 101 level and work our way to the 401 level - which covers the macronutrient view.

What all health coaching programs should teach you about nutrition: Nutrition 101 Water - Amount of water to drink is unique to everyone - Your body will adjust Basic Nutritional Concepts - Blood sugar, vitamins, minerals - Hydration and its importance Diets to review: Diets and what popular/negative impact they have in common media and wellness/pop culture Vegan Vegetarian Mediterranean Atkins Ohhh - don't forget, if it fits your macros, raw food, keto, WFPB, etc. Supplements - Research and regulatory - Advice for clients Nutrition and its impact on health coaches - Educating clients on micromovement to be effective - Emotional aspect of food - Nutrition of the inter-workings of our gut - Share amount of macronutrient science conducting into nutrition

Some clients are very interested in all of the "things" that we learn. However, most are interested in nutrition and heightening their nutrition literacy - so that is our primary goal. Nutrition and dietary guidelines are really important since what we put into our bodies has a huge impact on our lives and the quality of life we lead. For me, diet was the first domino that needed to fall in a quest to become a healthier, happier individual. Because nutrition is so huge, we must first find a way to make it easiest to consume and digest.

Basic Nutritional Concepts

Nutritional concepts need to be understood by a health coach in order to address the dietary needs and motivations of a client/patient. Physiology should be studied in general so that one can understand special nutritional conditions in various diseases, active states, and more. By gaining a good understanding of generally healthy mechanics and processes, it will be easier to assist in identifying and preparing interventions for when these processes break down or become imbalanced due to other factors.

SUBCUTANEOUS TISSUE Fat provides energy plus some vitamins. It insulates against heat loss and provides padding for vital parts. It is only recommended to store 7% body fat in men and 11% in women. Fat is the only nutrient that is completely lipophilic. Because the food we eat is often filled with toxins and hormones and other chemicals, the excess will be stored in our fat. This is why losing weight must be done slowly. If large amounts of fat are lost too quickly, the toxins will be dumped into the blood and can cause dizziness or even death. We should have twice as many Omega-6 fats in our bodies as Omega-3 fats. Americans have a 10 to 1 ratio.

FIBROUS TISSUE Fiber is also known as the bulky tissue. It plumps up with water and can range from watery to solid. Because it doesn't get digested, it helps to scrape the colon clean as it moves through. The average person should have 2 to 4 bowel movements a day in order to be healthy. Constipation is not simply an absence of bowel movements; it is a condition in which bowel movements are hard to pass. Only plants have fiber. Fiber draws cholesterol (a thick oil) out of arteries, and is beneficial in managing diabetes by slowing down the release of sugar from complex carbohydrates into the circulatory system, thereby avoiding blood sugar surges. A balanced amount of sugar will boost our metabolism, but too much can overwhelm the pancreas, which will have a hard time spitting out all the insulin needed.

Popular Diets and Their Impact

When working with clients, it is important to have a solid understanding of various dietary approaches so that you can help clients sift through the white noise and diet culture fads. Each diet has its merit and can be a good fit, depending on the consumer. Below are some of today's popular diets, in no particular order.

Keto Diet: The ketogenic diet is a low-carb, high-fat diet that results in a metabolic state called ketosis. When hormones are balanced and ketosis is reached, the body becomes ultra-efficient at burning fat for energy.

Paleo Diet: The theory behind the Paleo Diet is that by eating in a manner similar to our hunter-gatherer ancestors, we lower our risk of developing heart disease, cancer, diabetes, and other chronic diseases.

Thrive Diet: The Thrive Diet is a whole food, plant-based way of eating that leaves you feeling full and ready to tackle whatever comes your way.

Whole30: Whole30 is a month-long "reset" diet that allows only whole foods, no dairy, sugars of any kind, alcohol, grains, legumes, and processed foods. The idea is to reset something in our body such as hormone levels or our relationship with food.

FODMAP Diet: The low FODMAP diet essentially eliminates fermentable carbohydrates that are commonly malabsorbed in those with IBS or IBS-like conditions. This diet is considered better than a traditional IBS diet because it shows a decent amount of evidence and it works in the short-term to address certain aspects of IBS.

And many more.

4

Exercise and Fitness Programs

The purpose of this chapter is to:

    a. Help you understand the many dimensions of health and the role that physical activity plays in overall health;

    b. Discuss various types of physical activity: cardiovascular, strength and flexibility, and how each can be designed to meet your clients' needs;

    c. Summarize the benefits that your clients can derive from fitness programs;

    d. Provide recommendations for designing fitness programs - specifically, a format and exercises for each of the dimensions of physical activity (cardio, strength and flexibility).

The term "fitness" carries a lot of baggage. For some people, it refers to the shape they used to be in, while others will point to local health club excesses. Nevertheless, fitness does have some specific, generally accepted components and descriptions. In this chapter, fitness is described as the sum of the following three components: flexibility, strength, and cardiovascular (CV) endurance. CV endurance is synonymous with the term "aerobic endurance," but CV endurance also includes the energy systems used in longer weight training sessions. Rest is hard work, because it is production and recycling of energy. A default program for growth and repair, it only corresponds to good health and fitness if when the body is at rest, it recovers efficiently and effectively. In other words, the rest is simply a more passive or, better put, background process of producing and recovering from work. Since metabolic diseases take decades to develop, generally, and they usually result from patterns of diet and exercise (or inactivity), the overall framework for preventing and treating them includes physical as well as nutritional and emotional balance. Therefore, researchers and health professionals will need to give more attention to the effects of physical activity on health. We are health coaches, and part of our mission is to recommend exercise as much as proper healthy nutrition.

Types of Exercise and Their Benefits

Running isn't everything. It might be your favorite way to move, but are you doing a disservice to your health by pounding the pavement? That's a variable question. The type of exercise you do should be individual to you and your optimal health. People have been discussing the benefits of exercise for centuries. By combining routes, people can personalize their fitness program to maximize the benefits they want to obtain. With knowledge and expertise, your fitness coach can help you build your own fitness plan that's right for your body's unique needs and provide you customized health information.

In integrative health, we talk about four different types of exercise, and each of them comes with their own benefits. Exercise types include endurance/aerobic, strength, flexibility, balance and stability training. Many people who start exercise mainly want to change their body, weight, or muscle mass, but don't look only at the external benefits of a workout. To achieve optimal health, the network, as well as the health coach, needs to incorporate the whole body: body, mind, and spirit. It is not only the activity itself but also the environment in which physical activity occurs. Electromagnetism such as fitness center area, body of mind, type of activity and the type of people who attend the class include crucial variables. Eventually, everything irrespective of the kind of exercise, must be particular to you and your time. Thus, to enhance a fitness plan for you, focus on developing a bond relationship with a coach- a successful gym buddy. A fitness coach who can help you adjust your workout habits with superior benefits on mental and health and thus can be very helpful.

Designing Effective Fitness Programs

Before diving into the in-depth and strategic solutions for fitness program design, here are some informed tips and tricks to elevate the impact of the program and to contextually meet the immediate demands of the trainee.

Short answer quiz: any effective fitness program

The tight bent hinge at the waist is a very warm-up/stretch to prep for a big lift, like the RDL. Fiction Non-fiction Excessive ankle dorsiflexion and hip flexion should be corrected with a lifting shoe. Fiction Non-fiction Another name for a Landmine Press is a Meadows Row. Fiction Non-fiction Supine bridges help teach and isolate hip extension. Fiction Non-fiction The most global progression of the deadlift is the RDL, which requires the most loading. Fiction Non-fiction

The corrective exercise myth through the experience of Movement Debrief

Mythbusters Episode 792: Joseph Smith

Research with research showing that people simply love to read self-interested topics, therefore to make you interested in self-interest, there is research to back this research demonstrating that you are likely interested in this research. Sounds like an Onion article, doesn't it? Whether or not that's true, my interest here is in shedding light on the basic elements that closely relate to who we are and why we do what we do as fitness professionals. The fact that you are possibly interested in me saying this goes to show that humans are inherently self-concerned. Identifying this truth is the first step to understanding how to build killer sales leads for trainers in the fitness business. Knowing this, it seems self-evident that a great trainer would/should customize talking points in all sales pitches. It is a waste of time to dive into generalized service offerings because that's not what it's about. It is better to spend your time on personal experiences that are hypothetical for those you offer them.

5

Stress Management Techniques

According to the World Health Organization, stress is the "health epidemic of the 21st century." A Gallup poll found that 79% of Americans felt stress "frequently or sometimes." Long-term mild-to-moderate stress increases inflammation, suppresses immune function, increases the risk of chronic disease, impairs mental function, and disrupts sleep. Stress also contributes to food cravings and increased energy intake, especially energy-dense, palatable, high-sugar, high-fat snack foods, which can contribute to the proverbial "stress eating" and subsequent weight gain.

Effective mind-body stress relief practices such as mindfulness and meditation not only help regulate cortisol and sympathetic nervous system activity, they also increase resilience to stress. Researchers have found that people who practice mindfulness techniques for at least eight weeks are better able to cope with stress, that is, their cortisol levels normalize faster compared to those who do not practice mindfulness. In addition, meditation can shift brain activity. Researchers found that the more mindful people were, the less their brain activity in the amygdala, the brain's "fight or flight" center which mediates fear and anxiety.

Deep breathing exercises also help manage stress. They make you feel energized and alert. Breathing exercises have been shown to impact the parasympathetic nervous system, with the effects of these exercises differing depending on the length and timing of breath in relation to exhalation. Key points of the discussion with clients: Techniques that help people relax and calm their mind bring the body's stress response down, which has a positive impact on the immune system, inflammation, mental performance, and sleep. If someone is "in a flare," it is not the time to add a new stress-relief practice. Start with and experiment with a technique that helps them relax and feels like something they can maintain.

Mindfulness and Meditation

Mindfulness seems like the buzzword of the 21st century. And yet, this age-old practice of living in the moment continues to impact lives everywhere, including our personal health and wellness. The idea of mindfulness as a discrete concept emerged from the Buddhist practice of meditation, which has been undertaken for thousands of years. Modern research has shown that regularly practicing mindfulness can be tightly linked to our health, leading to reduced instances of stress, anxiety, depression, and disease. By allowing us to be conscious of our thoughts and emotions, practice acceptance, and take control of the way we react to stressors, mindfulness promotes mental and emotional health. As research progresses, we learn more about the benefits of mindfulness and how it contributes to overall well-being.

One of the most valuable things about learning the evidence-based science behind mindfulness is that you will then be able to confidently offer these researched, evidence-based techniques to others. The connection between stress and illness is laced with layers of myth, misinformation, and media hype, but that does not mean mental health is removed from wellness! On the contrary, practicing mindfulness is a vital, often untapped way of improving one's overall wellness and disease risk. Mindfulness and meditation have been proven to be effective tools in managing stress and improving various states of health and disease. Many people still think of meditation as one of those fringe wellness practices: sure, it's a nice idea, if only I had time. However, increasing evidence has shown that regular meditation practice can help improve your focus, psychological well-being, and even bodily health.

Breathing Exercises

There are a wide variety of breathing exercises. Here are a few that you might help recommend to your clients as starting points for those who want a quick relaxation in the middle of the work day or to help take a breather from stress. Remember to customize according to their goals and motivation for the most impact on behavior change - variety and relevance is key: DEA BREATH. Diaphragm exercise ensures they are engaging in a lung expanding breath and breathing fully to encourage relaxation.

Ask them to place their palm on their chest and the other on their abdomen. Tell them that when they take a deep breath in, the hand that is on the abdomen should rise higher than the one that is on the chest. DEEP SIX. Ask your client to breathe in for six long, slow seconds and exhale for six long, slow seconds to encourage the body to take energy-generating oxygen to the cells more efficiently and shift to relaxation mode. For those able to put their arms above their shoulders (this might not be everyone and if not, skip this), bring the arms into the air on the inhale and slowly back down to gently lift stress. In addition to breathing exercises, there are other stress management techniques that coaches may employ in their own lives or recommend to clients.

6

Client Assessment and Goal Setting

Great health practitioners seek to partner with their clients and encourage them through goal setting and goal achievement. Effective health coaches need the skill to assess their client's needs and resources, including their motivation level, and then help their client develop the skills they need to be successful. What strategies can we use to help us understand our client's needs and resources? The main tool we use is a health-risk assessment (HRA). HRAs have been used in worksite wellness programs for 30-40 years. Currently, questionnaires can be easily accessed online with a quick internet search for health-risk assessments. The HRA is designed to assess possible health risks, with the client's permission, and to assess the client's readiness to change, motivation to improve, knowledge, and confidence (or self-efficacy).

Questions must be followed by "The Confidence Scale, such as how confident are you that you could eat 3-4 cups of vegetables each day?" A score of 7-10 equals high self-efficacy, a score of 4-6 equals moderate self-efficacy, and a score of 1-3 equals low self-efficacy. This provides insight for the coach on where to start educating and increasing self-efficacy for their client. Health Coaches should make sure to assess their client's perception of their health; to not just rely on the cumulative score (quantitative data) but to interpret what that number means. After being assessed by an HRA, the coach and the client can establish goals that both the coach and the client believe are achievable. A well understood process to increase success in goal setting is the usage of the "SMART" acronym for clients: Specific, Measurable, Achievable, Realistic, and Timed. Clients who set SMART goals have an easier time being accountable for them and ultimately achieving them.

Assessment Tools and Techniques

Assessment tools and techniques. Health and wellness assessment provides an in-depth analysis of a client's status and needs. This thorough evaluation assists in the determination of the best route of care and therapeutics. The main purpose of an assessment is to provide a detailed snapshot of a client's current health and wellness status. This may include an assessment of all the factors that influence health and wellness such as physical, mental, emotional, environmental, occupational, and spiritual health/emotional health.

'Indirect' physical and health status assessments require extensive health history taking, lifestyle reviews, observation of habits/postures or living/working space set up. Information gathered from this assessment gives a provider a baseline of where the client currently is in terms of their health. This information will help to determine which treatment protocols will be most appropriate and also serves as a tool to reassess that client's health and success after a period of time. It helps to determine which therapeutics will be the most appropriate for the situation, as well as tracking the positive health and therapeutic outcomes.

Setting SMART Goals

Setting specific, measurable, achievable, relevant, and time-bound (SMART) goals can facilitate the well-being of the result expected from the wellness goal. The goal directs the development of targeted strategies to achieve a desired outcome rather than irrelevant goals which in themselves will not report wellness. Strategies assist in establishing measures needed to embody a "health story" to reach the desired wellness outcome.

Health coaching assists clients in facilitating the desire to recreate an improved personal wellness profile. The health coach assists the client one step beyond the mindset of being physically well as their client becomes motivated to experiencing high-quality energy which allows greater productivity in life. Setting personal wellness goals can be broken down into the developer strategies which proactively outline the direction required to achieve the desired outcome of the wellness profile. It is advised that the client measure the efforts exhibited in developing new strategies in order to see the desired outcome encapsulated in the wellness profile. The following table assists the development of the health story and consists of characteristics and definitions of each aspect. The client is directed in highlighting the various components as the 6 characteristics must be intertwined – if one of the characteristics is in isolation this will complicate the wellness story and thus personality wellness profile as a whole.

7

Communication and Coaching Skills

The success of a health coach hinges upon her ability to help clients help themselves. This begins with listening well, which is more than just being quiet or eagerly awaiting one's turn to speak. This kind of writing is also known as active listening. You also need perceptive or empathic listening, which is about identifying and validating the feelings behind what your client says, whether or not their emotions are explicit. Integrated wellness health coaches may ask clarifying questions, repeat advice in their own language, mirror a person's style of speech, or create metaphors to establish rapport.

The successful individual pursuing a career in integrated wellness should be someone who has strong empathy and listening skills, is culturally sensitive and open-minded with sound interpersonal abilities. Along with these empathetic traits, professionals should have a high level of intrinsic motivation, be resilient and persistent self-starters who are patient and have strong self-regulation and self-management. This kind of multicultural competence and emotional intelligence will help you connect with clients or patients on a more personal and effective level. In addition, the health coaching program is designed to provide individuals with the ability to begin their careers as health coaches in a variety of integrated wellness settings. You need strong oral and written communication skills to be able to motivate your clients and assist them in reaching their goals, in addition to your interpersonal skills. This includes creating relationships of trust with your clients as well as the other professionals you interact with and can include having the ability to share your own personal story in order to inspire change in your clients.

Active Listening

Active listening is a fancy way of saying, "really listen; pay attention." This might seem, at first glance, diminishing given the fact that the coaching course you are attending, Health & Wellness, involves coaching. However, human communication is so impaired due to the fact that we do not actually stop what we are doing to really listen to what the other person is saying. Current social dynamics shine with smartphones, which only enhance our incapacity for proper dialogue. If you want to be an effective coach, a competent coach, then active listening is more than an asset. It is an essential skill for understanding the client from their own perspective. Most people are exposed to at least some form of communication whereby they come away with the feeling that the other person did not really grasp what they wanted. It is frustrating and can build barriers between people.

Active listening involves total concentration on the part of the listener with as little interference as possible, both mental and physical. From a mental aspect, we would be discussing closely related concepts such as psychosomatics and psychoneuroimmunology. Physically, we are in fact referring to the environment of the clients and the coaching venue, but also to any interruptions, phone calls, unexpected visits, etc. Active listening, therefore, involves controlling all distractions and focusing your attention on what the client is saying. Specific attention is given to body language to pick up on unspoken dialogues, which (usually) can be heavy with emotions and laden with hidden clues. As a coach, you will need a good set of micro-skills – which we learned in the first module, Competent Communication.

Empathy and Building Rapport

Ultimately, coaching relies heavily upon the establishment of supportive connections between coach and client. Rapport in coaching has been defined as "a deep feeling of trust and camaraderie." This underpins every conversation and interaction that occurs under the omens of the coaching process. Rapport thus increases the coach's awareness of meaningful verbal and non-verbal signals, allowing them to connect as individuals while looking for potential leverage points in the coachee's resource base in order to support their individual pathway to success. Empathy is also a fundamental concept in coaching and has many definitions: coaches have been referred to as "outrageously pro-phone empathic," while the practice has been described as an emotional bridge in the coaching relationship, drawing upon sensitive communication and ensuring that "coaching is done with you rather than to you."

Generating this quality of rapport and empathy does require coaching to build their repertoire of communication skills and rely upon a number of change facilitation skills in order to manipulate or enhance the client's capacity to utilize desire, emotion, nutrition, and lifestyle to unleash the amazing adaptive resilience which is unique to living systems. This approach reinforces the idea that health coaching operates as an avenue for better enabling lifestyle interventions, thus allowing hard outcomes to match the intellectual ideal of promoting health in practice.

8

Ethical and Legal Considerations

During an initial session, openly discuss ethical and legal considerations. Stress that while confidentiality will be important, you may need to consult with other trusted professionals for appropriate referral and treatment. Reiterate your privacy policy. Touch base about boundaries. Clarify Recovery Coach and Health Coach roles and the preventive and lifestyle health coaching boundaries. Discourage disclosure of personal recovery status to clients. Present the scope of coaching. Make sure clients understand coaching is not therapy and is not appropriate for those needing psychological or psychiatric care. Explain and stress the risks and the unpredictable outcomes. Provide resources for further study.

It is important to uphold ethical standards while adhering to the legal framework in which your practice is located. The scope of practice varies from state to state in the United States with different regulations and requirements depending upon where an individual desires to practice. Additionally, if someone desires to accept insurance as a form of payment, they need to understand additional laws and regulations for insurance billing and compliance. The scope of practice standards varies by geographic location, such as state, country, or federal entity. Call or consult the regulatory board, such as the department of health, of the state or country in which an individual would like to practice for specific information about practice regulations. The focus here is on the United States of America. Review the American Medical Association's scope of practice and standards of practice policies with your clients. The AMA provides a general description of professional standards of practice. It outlines the educational requirements and certification for integrative wellness coaches. It also discusses the utilization of confidential information, the client's right to self-determination, and the importance of treating each client as a person.

Confidentiality and Boundaries

You motivate and enable a client to set goals and help your clients achieve results, focusing on nourishment and lifestyle. By doing so, however, practitioners have the right to know the limits and expectations of each profession. Health coaches should always understand confidentiality and professional boundaries in order to greatly reinforce responsibilities and obligations for practitioners. You will not offer assistance from a psychotherapist or medical professional as a professional, but curiosity is common.

Confidentiality is demonstrated through certain ethical standards for confidentiality. For instance, the Code of Ethics and Professional Standards has restricted access to client information for the International Association of Health Coaches. Standards also need to be set in relation to the limits, when what the client speaks with can not be said or shared. It's a fair guess with data on the special people mentioned during the session, because you'll be sharing a lot of people stories. Finally, a Health Coach may require a person's permission before sharing the specifics of their incidents and health history to the relevant authority. Often, the health coach has to clarify that these boundaries must be kept, but the ultimate aim is to empower the client to share—in words they have chosen for themselves—with those individuals who support them.

Scope of Practice

Health coaching has emerged as a distinct practice in healthcare within the wider continuum of wellness-driven care. Education and licensure as a health coach hold an individual to a certain standard of professional conduct and include the knowledge base necessary to work with clients in an effective and integral manner. How a health coach delivers services is delineated in the following text and serves as a source of guidance during health coaching encounters. Several health coaching methods are described below and indicate the working knowledge and understanding that individuals have when working with clients. Introduction to Health Coaching encompasses the biopsychosocial aspects of individual functioning and addresses the necessary competencies to help optimize health and wellness as a profession.

The erudition of health coaching theory, or foundation as it is called here, allows the coach a base from which to work. Education as a health coach is integral in granting the professional an understanding of the boundaries with which they function and the standards and guidelines under which they are to adhere. Working under specific guidelines is called hygiene, which relates to the nuts and bolts of the practice. As with any health profession, adherence to ethical standards is important. This centers on the idea of nonmaleficence, or the commitment to "do no harm" to the patient. Often these concepts are learned at the university level, granting foundational knowledge. However, many health professions require continuing education, which amounts to ongoing study in the field in order to keep personal growth in the practice. This "real world" experience is often gained through internships as well as on-the-job experience. However, educational modalities have only recently entered academic settings. A set of working competencies is indicated next, guiding both the everyday working health coach and providing support for instructors in increasing their depth of knowledge.

9

Business and Marketing Strategies

Building a successful health coaching practice involves business skills, marketing knowledge, and a good understanding of social media platforms and other resources. In this section, we will touch on the essentials of marketing, promotion, and content development for a health coaching business.

No matter what type of yoga teacher training or health coach certification you decide to pursue, the most important ability is business acumen and knowing how to market yourself. To build a successful health coaching practice, it's essential to know how to market your offerings correctly. Setting up a new website or sending out permission marketing emails requires a strategic approach as well as understanding the type of communication that is concise, compelling, and benefits-oriented. Using marketing to gently nudge potential clients to take action without applying pressure can turn those people into clients.

At the heart of digital marketing is creating a compelling presence online. This starts with creating useful and valuable content. Health coaches can share blog posts, podcast episodes, articles, or other resources that resonate most with their unique audiences. Following a thought leadership model, they can share what they know to be true and useful. They can provide easy-to-consume and actionable pieces of information, all while building up a profile or set of followers, and diving deeper into different topics through online courses. Every piece of content a health coach creates and shares is, in a way, a leading energy or leading conversation. It shows potential clients what they are about and delivers on what they promise.

Setting Up Your Health Coaching Practice

To help you begin translating the experience and skills you've developed in your Integrative Nutrition Health Coach Training Program into a professional practice, we have developed 4 roadmaps that you may use in whole, or in part, to guide you through the process. First, we have a business development guide that you may use to begin formulating your business plan and operational system. The second guide is the third set of questions to help you clarify your business goals, mission, and message. We then have two plans, one for setting up a private coaching practice, and one for setting up a group practice. We hope this will help to move you in the direction you envision most.

The keys to success in leading any business are to be prepared, be passionate, find an underserved, viable market, and to take small, effective steps toward that market. This business development guide was created by well-known business coach and Integrative Nutrition faculty Rick Jarow, PhD. Within these pages, he covers all of the basic issues you will need to address as you begin to create and organize your thoughts about starting a health coaching business. This guide is not completely comprehensive, nor does it cover many of the complex business development issues an entrepreneur will face. It gives you a place to begin. At any point during your brainstorming, you should also consult with financial, legal, or general consultants for their expert advice, and companion guides to set up your professional practice.

Attracting and Retaining Clients

The strategies you employ for attracting clients are the same strategies you'll use to keep those clients and create a long-term relationship. You won't want to be constantly scrambling for new clients; it's better to retain existing clients and add new ones as time goes on. Here are a few key techniques to keep in mind when trying to retain clients.

Use your marketing materials. Your website, email campaigns, e-books, and white papers shouldn't just be used for attracting new clients, they should also be used for retaining them. Keep clients coming back for more by sending them regular updates, newsletters outlining your latest ideas, and quick tips.

Follow up on unfinished business. A client who fails to sign on with you is simply showing a lack of commitment and readiness at the time you approach them. Keep in touch in a genuine way by sending them additional free material, useful articles, or information on your practice, and encourage them to pick a date for a second free sample session in the future. They may be ready another day, and you could have another client!

Promote a free or reduced-rate program for friends. Let your current clients know that your practice is growing and that you have openings for a scaled-down program for those close to them, such as friends and associates. Offer them a discount to give to friends for a free or $20 session. If their friend signs up for the comprehensive program, discount their own program by $100.

10

Case Studies and Practical Applications

Excerpt number 10 focuses on a diverse array of practical, real-life client scenarios, as well as applications situated in the reality of the workplace. Each case study summarizes the presenting issues, client history or background, how each health coach used the relevant core concepts and what recommendations they made to their client, and finally the outcome. Each practical application illustrates real-world use of the same theory and concepts in a work-setting or with clients.

Case Studies

Case study 1: Healthy mothers = healthy children. Theory and application: Grounding, listening, being present and connected to the teachings of the past. Recommendations: Stick to the basics, go to bed early, eat lots of green leafy vegetables and slow-digesting fermented foods. Outcome: Re-evaluation – no changes to client scenarios.

Case study 2: A taste of Thailand. Theory and application: The need for contextual understanding in the coaching conversation. Recommendations: Focus on quality protein, 5+ serves of vegetables, 2 or 3 serves of low-GI carbs and a sugar 'cut-off'. Outcome: Re-evaluation – diet modification and decreased caffeine intake.

Case study 3: The hard-eating ex-vegetarian. Theory and application: The need for balance and homeostasis. Recommendations: Focus on whole, fresh, local, unprocessed foods that are as close to natural as possible. Outcome: Further testing required.

Case study 4: Sarah. Theoretically based applications: Initial strategy – Reduce psychological and emotional stress, begin an anti-inflammatory protocol, address dysbiosis/infection, develop dietary plan. Additional recommendations: Increase rest time, increase time in nature, begin a daily yoga practice, undertake quarterly short fasting for health. Outcome: Client is currently undergoing parasitology testing. Anxiety levels have dramatically reduced, and Sarah has been able to resume a healthy diet.

Practical Applications.

Practical Application 1: Offering a Lunch and Learn session on 'Eating for Stress' in the workplace.

Practical Application 2: Establishing a volunteer, client-centred health coaching service in the student clinic of a natural medicine college.

Real-Life Client Scenarios

Developing and implementing a coaching business can be more fully understood and integrated through experience with real-life client scenarios. A number of true-to-life coaching situations will be offered to highlight how you might apply the theoretical information gained through your wellness coach experience. Hopefully, this will provide more information to build greater confidence in working with more diverse clients in a broader context. Each case scenario concludes with some fundamentals that would be useful to consider when contemplating coaching each individual. Case scenarios include clients looking for help with stress, weight, sugar cravings, exercise, personal development, self-care, nutrition, food shopping, career change, and supplementation.

The case scenarios are based on coaching sessions conducted at the Arizona Center for Integrative Medicine's two-week Intensive Skills Workshop, which is an elective for students in the Integrative Wellness Coaching (IWC) course. The IWC is an approved grandfathered health and wellness coach training program by the National Consortium for Credentialing Health and Wellness Coaches. This integrative coaching program is grounded in positive psychology and culminates in an 80-hour certificate of completion. The experiential scenarios of 80 low-income volunteers interested in making significant lifestyle changes were graduated by 21 wellness coach students. Each student conducted multiple sessions for 3 to 4 of the volunteers and kept a daily journal that outlined the intention of the session, responses, observations, and lessons learned each time the volunteers completed assessments. Sessions included goal setting, partnership building, stakeholders and determinants of change identification, refining heart and smart goals, personalized alternative track creation on all assessment findings, self-responsibility and self-efficacy activities, and finally a group options and expectations activity.

Applying Integrative Wellness Principles

What good is it to understand wellness promotion and positive health strategies if you cannot translate them into meaningful client interactions? Let's review how the principles of integrative wellness may be used in your role as a health coach.

Fundamental is the fact that integrative wellness is an important and valuable alignment to health coaching and coaching in general. The prominence of integrative wellness principles offers a way for coaches to intersect philosophy, theory, and practical application by focusing on a greater goal of optimal physiological balance, energy, and resilience. The practical applications of integrative wellness principles are both simple and complex. Interactions depend not just on the idea but the audience and the environment where they are offered. There is individualization to consider, such as engagement in a bariatric surgery population versus a group of relatively healthy individuals. Thinking about ways we can put these principles into action may require consideration of individual or group workshops, individual behavior change strategies, stress management class structure, and many other "real-life" contexts. Here are five steps that might help you begin thinking about how to bring integrative wellness principles into your coaching.

11

Continuing Education and Professional Development

A dvanced Certification Opportunities
Many integrative medicine post-graduate training programs offer some type of certification in health coaching. Other institutes and programs provide certificates that are intended as credentials. The actual name of the title, such as Certified Health, Wellness, or Wellness Inventory Coach, is unique to each program. We do not intend, or imply any endorsement by including them here. These institutes and their programs are listed in alphabetical order.

Center for Integrative Medicine Program in Integrative Health at the University of Arizona (AzCIM/PihH) in Tucson, Arizona. The Center for Mind-Body Medicine Professional Training Program: Food as Medicine, Mind, Body, Environment, Spirit in Washington, D.C. and around the country. Duke Integrative Medicine Duke Coaching Skills Trainings in Durham, North Carolina. Integrative Nutrition in Washington, D.C. and New York, N.Y. offers a one-year course on nutrition and coaching. Nutrition Therapy Institute in Denver, Colo. offers a course in functional nutrition and holistic chef. University of Minnesota Center for Spirituality & Healing in

Minneapolis, Minnesota. Whitney Center is based in Fairfax, Massachusetts. It offers a presentation called "Turn-ons and Turn-offs: Nutrition and Obesity Solutions for Integrative Practitioners".

Special Advanced Workshop and Retreat Offerings

Additional workshops and retreats are being held in Wisconsin this fall, and in Germany and New Zealand in the fall and winter. The goals of these workshops and retreats are to enable people to learn whether or not health coaching is a practice they want to establish and to enable them to learn the different ways they might integrate health coaching into their present and future practices. Discussing the world of whole health and healthcare informatics just show the depth to which we must educate our clients in many domains.

Certifications and Credentials

Certifications are available from various organizations, but the most respected certification is the National Board for Health & Wellness Coaching (NBHWC). Starting in November 2017, the NBHWC began certifying health & wellness coaches. The process is rigorous and requires 60 hours of approved coach training and completion of a final exam. Health coaches have the option to further enhance their qualifications. For example, students can pursue a National Commission for Health Education Credentialing (NCHEC) certification in health education. Additionally, in some of the programs discussed above, RD's may pursue a Board Certified-Advanced Diabetes Management (BC-ADM). Personal trainers and group fitness instructors also have pursued various credentials from the American College of Sports Medicine and other organizations.

Students will receive all of the nutrition and wellness coach training necessary to become a successful health coach and educator. Students are then ready to take the IIN (Integrated Institute of Nutrition) final exam and become a board certified health and wellness coach. The FMCA will then provide 40 hours of practical experience including client coaching and/or group coaching throughout the internship period. When students become a qualified health and wellness coach, they then have the option of staying on as a contracted coach with the FMCA and continuing to work with clients and/or groups under the guidance of the FMCA team. This credential demonstrates the highest level of experience, expertise, and credibility a professional health coach in the field possesses.

Workshops and Seminars

Completion of workshops and seminars related to health and wellness-related professional development is a great way to add to your current knowledge base and show a willingness to stay updated with industry trends. Unlike certificate programs, workshops/seminars typically require 1 to 3 days and may or may not result in an actual "certificate." Sometimes the training is more experiential rather than academic, so plan to choose training opportunities that will fit with your personal learning style and/or how you best learn and grow professionally. Choose trainings that are meaningful for you, fit with your personal and professional values, and will help you to demonstrate to your clients that you offer them the best because you continue to strive for the best in yourself. Include certifications and/or licenses as well as any workshops/seminars that you have attended and are incomplete.

Nothing says "the best coach" quite like a commitment to continuous and dynamic professional development. There is one truth to health and wellness: it's always changing. If you are looking for ways to continue growing as a Medicine Coach and gain insight into new industry trends, look into possibilities in the following areas of interest. Keep reading for organizations across the nation that offer fantastic learning opportunities! Please note: Some of these education programs are not directly related to health coaching. Many of these offerings do, however, have significant relevance to the development of an integrative wellness coaching approach.

12

Conclusion and Future Trends

Twelve modules and many chapters later, you have begun your Integrative Nutrition health coaching journey. We hope that this comprehensive guide to the field has opened a myriad of possibilities for you and awoken that fiery passion you have within. Becoming a health coach is an active and ongoing process, and not simply a destination to reach. By exploring the foundations of wellness, focusing on your personal and professional success, and delving into principles of coaching, it is our hope that you have become not only more knowledgeable and perceptive about your own life, but also ways in which to work with your future clients. This guide has been crafted in a way that can become a stepping stone to your future, a future full of positivity and shifting paradigms.

If we had written this book many years in the past or to a future audience, there would be a few dates and chapters that would be different. The world of integrative wellness is a delicate and ever-evolving field. We can tell you, however, that trends are placing ever-increasing emphasis on innovation and how an integrative approach to wellness encompasses more than just food. And while today, in 2022 and beyond, it is important to remember the primary tenet of belief that went into you enrolling in this program and beginning this book: for countless reasons, food is much more than food. Next, let's look ahead to the future of our rapidly growing wellness land-scape. Designing buildings with health at the center, virtual reality bringing health and wellness services straight into your home, med-ical multidisciplinary research teams studying mind-body modalities in depth, and health coaching being covered by insurance and em-braced by corporations are some of the rapidly emerging trends we are beginning to see. And we expect, and work towards, to see even more movements just like these!

Reflecting on Your Health Coaching Journey

More and more primary care physicians are referring their pa-tients to health coaches. Many health coaches are making a living on their own and partnering with professionals across the health spec-trum to improve client outcomes. With the overwhelming central-formalized education dominating the airwaves, many individuals are turning to health coaching education for comprehensive programs in integrative and functional wellness. Reflecting on the path to be-coming a health coach may lead to introspection and self-assessment on what exactly it means to be a health coach. It may lead health pro-fessionals on a path they are yet to have journeyed upon. After com-pletion of a health coaching program, clinicians are restored with purpose and passion.

The pathway to health and wellness is arduous before one can be of service to others. Although, there appear to be health-related benefits to walking under arcades of leaves and alongside precious gurgling water. Peppering your trainings, trainings from or endorse-ments with individuals also build off the functional medicine par-adigm and many of us have trained with additional experts in their respective fields. These unique integrative wellness knowledge bases propel you forward in your life redesign journey. For very little extra time, you can arrange for these value-added bits of fabulosity. Actions begin by critically reflecting over the enlivening live modules you have been soaked in. The heaviness of the content is often accompanied by light, laughter and transformation that builds.

Emerging Trends in Integrative Wellness

Drawing upon key insights from health and wellness coach training (HWCT) providers' primary narrative data, this chapter explores emerging promising practices that providers are developing in response to today's rapidly transforming healthcare landscape. Through participatory input sessions conducted during cross-institutional conferences in March 2021 and August 2021, where a diverse group of HWCT providers shared, celebrated, and interrogated their own efforts and strategies, we identified opportunities that showcase the transformative power of coaching.

Diverging paths drawn from these sessions gave us a much clearer sense of emerging trends worth summarizing. In the disruptive grammar of today's health environment, integrative wellness and meaningful partnerships with people, individual or collective, on the healing journey are foundational. And as a result, new trends are forcing their way forward, forging transformational paths in our midst. We believe it will only behoove all of us to see and name these leading lights in the landscape so that we might learn from them or collaboratively bring them into fuller, brighter, integrate-able existence.

This rising chapter discusses developing themes while also reporting on the current state of our training activity, given the altered environment of 2020. In capturing principal themes from the Promising Practices session, it is our desire to bring clarity to our unfolding story, to honor our collective strengths, alignment, ambitions, and investment. While each session was standalone, and members came from different vantage points and worldview orientations, session leaders Jeff Rays and Heather Green lead the development of this article, with the entirety of this cross-institutional collaboration comprising Michele P. Robotham, Cory Lemoine, Gina Squis Worth, Sue Haskins, Moira Raphael, Lisa Morse, Heather Green, and Jeff Rays.